Gluten

Fast Food Restaurants

Adam Bryan

Published by Diamondhead Studios

First published in 2011

Menus updated in 2012

To you, my readers, and true supporters.

Thank you.

Acknowledgments

I would like to thank my friends and family for their support. And of course you the reader for reading my book. I truly do appreciate it.

Best wishes,

Adam Bryan
Author

Table of Contents

Introduction: What is Gluten?

The term "gluten" technically refers to a specific complex of proteins that forms when wheat flour is mixed with a liquid and physically manipulated, such as in the kneading of bread. The Food and Drug Administration (FDA) is proposing to define the term "gluten" to mean the proteins that naturally occur in a prohibited grain (see below) and that may cause adverse health effects in persons with celiac disease.

In a more simplified definition, gluten is what most scientists like to call a storage protein. Its what gives dough the elastic texture and feel to it. Prolamins are a class of proteins present in a variety of grains, and they're what cause problems for people who can't eat gluten. Gluten has become a more general term for any kind of potentially harmful prolamin. The prolamins that tend to cause damage to people with celiac disease or any other gluten allergies include gliadin, found in wheat, secalin, found in rye, and horedin, found in barley.

Popular Foods and Drinks that Contain Gluten

- ✘ Bagels
- ✘ Beer
- ✘ Bread
- ✘ Cereals (most contain gluten unless clearly noted "gluten-free" on the box)
- ✘ Cookies, cakes, most baked goods, and pastries
- ✘ Crackers
- ✘ Licorice
- ✘ Pasta
- ✘ Pizza
- ✘ Pretzels

A Gluten Free Life

As we all know, eating out at fast food establishments with celiac disease, gluten allergy, or even a special gluten-free diet can sometimes be very risky and stressful.

It's always a guessing game as to finding out if your food contains any traces of gluten unless you ask one of the workers at your dining establishment.

Well now you can eat with confidence thanks to the *Gluten-Free Guide to Fast Food Restaurants.*

In here, you will be provided with a comprehensive list of foods and drinks that you **can** enjoy at most popular fast food chains in the United States and even some internationally. From burgers and fries to seafood and frozen yogurt, this guide has them all.

Who would've thought eating out would be this easy!

Warning!

Although these restaurants provide gluten free menu items, they do encourage anyone with food sensitivities, allergies, or special dietary needs to consult with a medical professional for informed answers relating to their specific sensitivities and the risks involved when dining out. Also please be aware that some food will be in the presence of gluten items, such as in sandwich and delis, so please be advised and use caution.

Also, please be sure to talk alert the fast food restaurant that you have a gluten allergy so that they can take the proper measures. Thank you.

Burgers and Beef

Arby's

Meats

- ✓ Black Angus Roast Beef
- ✓ Corned Beef
- ✓ Genoa Salami
- ✓ Pecan Chicken Salad
- ✓ Pepper Bacon
- ✓ Pepperoni
- ✓ Roast Beef
- ✓ Roast Chicken
- ✓ Roast Ham Roast Turkey
- ✓ Sides
- ✓ Applesauce

Salads

- ✓ Chopped Farmhouse Salad-Turkey & Ham
- ✓ Chopped Farmhouse Chicken-Roast
- ✓ Chopped Side Salad

Condiments:

- ✓ Arby's Sauce
- ✓ Banana Peppers
- ✓ Chargrill Seasoning
- ✓ Cheddar Cheese Sauce+
- ✓ Cheddar Cheese, Sharp Natural Slice
- ✓ Cheddar Cheese, Shredded Natural

- ✓ Cheddar Cheese, Processed Slice
- ✓ Dijon Honey Mustard Sandwich Sauce
- ✓ Dill Pickle Slices
- ✓ Horsey Sauce
- ✓ Ketchup
- ✓ Mayonnaise
- ✓ Parmesan Peppercorn Ranch Sauce
- ✓ Pecan Chicken Salad
- ✓ Pepper & Onion Mix
- ✓ Red Ranch Sauce
- ✓ Red Wine Vinaigrette Sauce
- ✓ Sauerkraut
- ✓ Smoky Q Sauce
- ✓ Spicy Brown Honey Mustard Sauce
- ✓ Swiss Cheese, Big Eye Natural
- ✓ Swiss Cheese, Processed Slice
- ✓ Thousand Island Spread
- ✓ Yellow Mustard

Dressings

- ✓ Balsamic Vinaigrette Dressing
- ✓ Buttermilk Ranch Dressing
- ✓ Dijon Honey Mustard Dressing
- ✓ Light Italian Dressing

Dipping Sauces

- ✓ Buffalo Sauce
- ✓ Honey Dijon Mustard Sauce
- ✓ Ranch Sauce
- ✓ Tangy Barbeque Sauce

- ✓ Bronco Berry Sauce

Beverages

- ✓ 1% Low Fat Chocolate Milk
- ✓ 2% Reduced Fat Milk
- ✓ CapriSun Fruit Juice
- ✓ Coffee
- ✓ Diet Pepsi
- ✓ Dr Pepper
- ✓ Mountain Dew
- ✓ Pepsi
- ✓ Sierra Mist
- ✓ Brewed Iced Tea
- ✓ Nestlé Pure Life Bottled Water

Desserts

- ✓ Chocolate Shake
- ✓ Jamocha Swirl Shake
- ✓ Vanilla Shake

A&W

A&W restaurants won't recommend any of their meats or poultry products to those with Celiac disease, or gluten free diets because of common cooking equipment.

Toppings and Sauces

- ✓ Cheese

- ✓ Honey Mustard Dipping Sauce
- ✓ Ranch Dipping Sauce
- ✓ Papa Sauce
- ✓ Cheese Sauces

Sweets and Treats

- ✓ Reese's Polar Swirl
- ✓ Vanilla Milkshake
- ✓ Strawberry Milkshake
- ✓ Chocolate Milkshake
- ✓ Root Beer Freeze
- ✓ Root Beer Float
- ✓ Strawberry Sundae
- ✓ Hot Fudge Sundae
- ✓ Caramel Sundae

Boardwalk Fries

- ✓ French Fries cooked in gluten-free peanut oil

Burger King

Meats

- ✓ WHOPPER Patty
- ✓ WHOPPER JR. Patty
- ✓ Steakhouse XT™ Patty
- ✓ Hamburger Patty
- ✓ Bacon Slice
- ✓ Ham Slice
- ✓ TENDERGRILL Chicken Breast Filet

- ✓ Egg Omelet
- ✓ Tacos
- ✓ Sausage Patty

Sides
- ✓ BK Fresh Apple Fries
- ✓ Salad Mix
- ✓ French Fries

Toppings
- ✓ Lettuce
- ✓ Sliced Onions
- ✓ Carrots
- ✓ Sliced Tomato
- ✓ Sliced Pickle
- ✓ Processed American Cheese
- ✓ Processed Pepper Jack Cheese
- ✓ Processed Cheddar (Sharp)
- ✓ Processed Swiss Cheese
- ✓ Three-Cheese Blend

Sauces and Condiments
- ✓ BBQ Dipping Sauce
- ✓ Buffalo Dipping Sauce
- ✓ Stacker Sauce
- ✓ Smoky Cheese Sauce
- ✓ Caramel Sauce
- ✓ Chocolate Fudge Sauce
- ✓ Sweet and Sour Dipping Sauce
- ✓ French Fry Sauce
- ✓ Honey Mustard Dipping Sauce

- ✓ Marinara Sauce
- ✓ Ranch Dipping Sauce
- ✓ A.1. Thick and Hearty Steaksauce
- ✓ Sweet Baby Ray's Hot 'n Spicy BBQ Sauce
- ✓ Tartar Sauce
- ✓ Zesty Onion Ring Sauce
- ✓ Vanilla Icing
- ✓ KEN'S Honey Mustard, Light Italian, Ranch
- ✓ Breakfast Syrup
- ✓ Grape Jam
- ✓ Honey
- ✓ Ketchup
- ✓ Mustard
- ✓ Mayonnaise
- ✓ Strawberry Jam

Beverages

- ✓ Barq's Root Beer
- ✓ Frozen Coke
- ✓ Coca-Cola Classic
- ✓ Coca-Cola
- ✓ Diet Coke
- ✓ Dr. Pepper
- ✓ Sprite
- ✓ MINUTE MAID Lemonade
- ✓ MINUTE MAID 100% Apple and Orange Juice
- ✓ NESTLÉ PURE LIFE Purified Drinking Water
- ✓ Seattle's Best Coffee
- ✓ Fat-Free Milk
- ✓ 1% Lowfat Chocolate Milk

Desserts
- ✓ Chocolate, Vanilla and Strawberry Shakes
- ✓ Soft-Serve in a Cup

Carl's Jr

- ✓ Gluten-Sensitive - 1/3 lb. Low Carb Thickburger
- ✓ Gluten-Sensitive - Low Carb Breakfast Bowl
- ✓ Gluten-Sensitive - Side Salad

Culver's

Salads

- ✓ Chicken Cashew with Flame Roasted Chicken
- ✓ Cranberry Bacon Bleu Salad
- ✓ Strawberry Fields Salad
- ✓ Tossed Tuna Salad
- ✓ Tossed Chicken Salad

Dressings and Condiments

- ✓ All Condiments
- ✓ Caesar Dressing
- ✓ Chunky Bleu Cheese Dressing
- ✓ French Dressing
- ✓ French Dressing Reduced Calorie
- ✓ Ranch Dressing
- ✓ Ranch Dressing Reduced Calorie

Sides

- ✓ Crinkle Cut Fries
- ✓ Cole Slaw
- ✓ Green Beans
- ✓ Sweet Potato Fries

Soups

- ✓ Baja Chicken Enchilada
- ✓ Corn Chowder
- ✓ Mushroom Medley
- ✓ Potato Au Gratin

Desserts and Milkshakes

- ✓ Banana Split
- ✓ Caramel Cashew
- ✓ Fudge Pecan Sundae
- ✓ Turtle Sundae
- ✓ Vanilla Shake
- ✓ Chocolate Shake
- ✓ Culver's Root Beer Float
- ✓ Lemon Ice Cooler
- ✓ Lemon Ice Smoothie
- ✓ Mint Chip Shake
- ✓ Old Fashioned Cherry Soda
- ✓ Chocolate Dish
- ✓ Chocolate Frozen Custard
- ✓ Vanilla Dish
- ✓ Vanilla Frozen Custard
- ✓ Vanilla Concrete Mixer

- ✓ Chocolate Concrete Mixer
- ✓ Turtle Concrete Mixer

Hardees

- ✓ Gluten-Sensitive - 1/3 lb. Low Carb Thickburger
- ✓ Gluten-Sensitive - Low Carb Breakfast Bowl
- ✓ Gluten-Sensitive - Side Salad

Jack In the Box

Entrees

- ✓ Grilled chicken strips (4 pc)

Salads and Dressings

- ✓ Chicken Club Salad w/Grilled Chicken Strips
- ✓ Grilled Chicken Salad
- ✓ Side Salad
- ✓ Southwest Chicken Salad w/Grilled Chicken Strips
- ✓ Bacon Ranch Dressing
- ✓ Creamy Southwest Dressing
- ✓ Gourmet Seasoned Croutons
- ✓ Lite Ranch Dressing
- ✓ Low Fat Balsamic Vinaigrette Dressing
- ✓ Spicy Corn Sticks
- ✓ Hearty Breakfast Bowl

Sides

- ✓ Hashbrown Sticks (5 pc.)
- ✓ Chiquita® Apple Bites with caramel

Sauces and Condiments

- ✓ Barbecue Dipping Sauce
- ✓ Buttermilk House Dipping Sauce
- ✓ Fire Roasted Salsa
- ✓ Frank's®
- ✓ RedHot®
- ✓ Buffalo Dipping Sauce
- ✓ Honey Mustard Dipping Sauce
- ✓ Log Cabin®
- ✓ Syrup
- ✓ Sweet & Sour Dipping Sauce
- ✓ Tartar Sauce
- ✓ Zesty Marinara Sauce
- ✓ Substitute Sauces Allergens Soy Egg Fish Milk Peanuts
- ✓ Crustacean
- ✓ Shellfish Tree Nuts Wheat
- ✓ Chipotle Sauce
- ✓ Creamy Italian Sauce
- ✓ Creamy Ranch Sauce
- ✓ Ketchup
- ✓ Mayo-Onion
- ✓ Mustard
- ✓ Peppercorn Mayo
- ✓ Sun Dried Tomato Sauce

- ✓ Fire Roasted Salsa
- ✓ Grape Jelly
- ✓ Grilled Onions
- ✓ Ketchup
- ✓ Malt Vinegar
- ✓ Mayonnaise
- ✓ Mustard
- ✓ Pride Margarine Spread
- ✓ Red Onion
- ✓ Secret Sauce
- ✓ Sour Cream
- ✓ Strawberry Jelly
- ✓ Taco Sauce

Drinks and Beverages

- ✓ All drinks and beverages

Desserts

- ✓ Blackberry Shake with Whipped Topping
- ✓ Rootbeer Float
- ✓ Strawberry Shake with Whipped Topping
- ✓ Vanilla Shake with Whipped Topping

McDonalds

Meats
- ✓ Beef Patty (no bun)
- ✓ Breakfast Beef Steak

✓ Canadian Bacon
✓ Sausage
✓ Scrambled Egg

Sides

✓ Fruit 'n Yogurt Parfait (no granola)

McDonald's Salads/Dressings

✓ Caesar Salad w/o Chicken
✓ Side Salad
✓ Newman's Own Creamy Caesar Dressing
✓ Newman's Own Cobb Dressing
✓ Newman's Own Low Fat Balsamic Vinaigrette
✓ Newman's Own Ranch Dressing
✓ Newman's Own Salsa

Drinks, Beverages, and Desserts

✓ Apple Juice
✓ Coffee
✓ Hot Chocolate
✓ 1% Low Fat Milk, White or Chocolate
✓ Orange Juice
✓ Soft Drinks
✓ Chocolate Triple Thick Shake
✓ Strawberry Triple Thick Shake
✓ Vanilla Triple Thick Shake
✓ Ice Cream Sundaes including nuts
✓ McFlurry with M&M'S Candies

Sauces and Condiments

- ✓ Butter
- ✓ Chicken McNugget Honey
- ✓ Chicken McNugget Hot Mustard Sauce
- ✓ Hotcake Syrup
- ✓ Jam
- ✓ Ketchup
- ✓ Lettuce
- ✓ Margarine
- ✓ Mayonnaise
- ✓ Mustard
- ✓ Onions
- ✓ Pickles
- ✓ Tartar Sauce
- ✓ Tomato
- ✓ Apple Dippers and Low Fat Caramel Dip
- ✓ McDonald's Cheeses:
- ✓ American Cheese

Sonic

Grill Items

- ✓ Hamburger Patty
- ✓ Angus Burger with no bun
- ✓ Bacon
- ✓ Breakfast Sausage
- ✓ Hot Dog
- ✓ Steak
- ✓ Egg

Sides

- ✓ French Fries
- ✓ Tots
- ✓ Apple Slices

Cheese

- ✓ Sliced American Cheese
- ✓ Shredded Colby Jack Cheese
- ✓ Shredded Cheddar Cheese

Sauces and Condiments

- ✓ All Sandwich Sauces
- ✓ All Condiments

Shakes, Drinks, and Dessert Toppings

- ✓ Soft Serve (Vanilla)
- ✓ 1% Chocolate Milk
- ✓ 1% Milk
- ✓ Whipped Dessert Topping
- ✓ Butterfinger
- ✓ M&M's
- ✓ Reese's(R)
- ✓ Neutral Slush Base
- ✓ Cherry Syrup
- ✓ Low-Cal Diet Cherry Syrup
- ✓ Grape Syrup
- ✓ Blue Coconut Syrup
- ✓ Bubble Gum Syrup
- ✓ Orange Syrup

- ✓ Cream Pie Syrup
- ✓ Green Apple Syrup
- ✓ Watermelon Syrup
- ✓ Maraschino Cherries
- ✓ Pineapple Topping
- ✓ Strawberry Topping
- ✓ Caramel Topping
- ✓ Butterscotch
- ✓ Chocolate Syrup
- ✓ Peanut Butter Topping

Wendy's

Entrée

- ✓ Hamburger Patty
- ✓ Ultimate Chicken Grill Fillet

Baked Potatoes

- ✓ Plain
- ✓ Sour Cream & Chives
- ✓ Cheese
- ✓ Bacon & Cheese
- ✓ Broccoli & Cheese
- ✓ Chili & Cheese

Side Items

- ✓ Apple Slices
- ✓ Chili
- ✓ Hot Chili Seasoning Packet

- ✓ Cheddar Cheese, shredded

Frosty™

- ✓ Chocolate Frosty
- ✓ Vanilla Frosty
- ✓ Chocolate Frosty Shake
- ✓ Strawberry Frosty Shake
- ✓ Vanilla Bean Frosty Shake
- ✓ Wild Berry Frosty Shake
- ✓ Caramel Frosty Shake
- ✓ Caramel Apple Frosty Parfait (without granola)

Salads

- ✓ Caesar Side Salad (without croutons)
- ✓ Garden Side Salad (without croutons)
- ✓ Baja Salad
- ✓ Seasoned Tortilla Strips+
- ✓ Apple Pecan Chicken Salad (without pecans)
- ✓ BLT Cobb Salad

Dressings

- ✓ Avocado Ranch Dressing
- ✓ Classic Ranch Dressing
- ✓ Creamy Red Jalapeno Dressing
- ✓ Fat Free French Dressing
- ✓ Italian Vinaigrette Dressing
- ✓ Lemon Garlic Caesar Dressing

- ✓ Light Classic Ranch Dressing
- ✓ Pomegranate Vinaigrette Dressing
- ✓ Thousand Island Dressing

Sauce and Condiments

- ✓ American Cheese
- ✓ Applewood Smoked Bacon
- ✓ Buttery Best Spread
- ✓ Cheddar Cheese Sauce
- ✓ Dill Pickles
- ✓ Honey Mustard Sauce
- ✓ Ketchup
- ✓ Lettuce
- ✓ Mustard
- ✓ Mayonnaise
- ✓ Natural Asiago Cheese
- ✓ Cheddar & Pepper Jack Cheese Blend
- ✓ Red Onion
- ✓ Ranch Sauce
- ✓ Reduced Fat Sour Cream+
- ✓ Tomato
- ✓ Tartar Sauce

Beverages

- ✓ Coffee
- ✓ Coffee Creamer
- ✓ Iced Tea
- ✓ Hot Tea
- ✓ Sweet Tea
- ✓ Coca-Cola

- ✓ Diet Coke
- ✓ Sprite
- ✓ Barq's Root Beer
- ✓ Coke ZeroTM
- ✓ Dr Pepper
- ✓ Fanta Orange
- ✓ Hi-C Flashin' Fruit Punch
- ✓ Minute Maid Light Lemonade
- ✓ Pibb Xtra
- ✓ TruMoo Lowfat White Milk
- ✓ TruMoo Lowfat Chocolate Milk
- ✓ Nestlé Pure Life Bottled Water
- ✓ Juicy Juice Apple Juice
- ✓ Nestea Unsweetened Iced Tea
- ✓ Nestea Sweetened Iced Tea

White Castle

Entrees

- ✓ Chicken Rings
- ✓ Buffalo Chicken Rings
- ✓ Ranch Chicken Rings
- ✓ Clam Strips

Sides

- ✓ Mozzerella Cheese Sticks
- ✓ French Fries
- ✓ Cheese Fries
- ✓ Loaded Fries (cheddar and bacon)
- ✓ Loaded Fries (cheddar, bacon, and ranch)

- ✓ Loaded Fries (bacon and ranch)
- ✓ Sweet Potato Fries
- ✓ Onion Rings

Sauces and Condiments

- ✓ All side sauces except Ranch
- ✓ All sauces and condiments

Beverages

- ✓ All beverages including coffee

Desserts

- ✓ Apple Turnovver
- ✓ Brach's Fruit Orchard Snack
- ✓ Chocolate Chip Cookie
- ✓ Oatmeal Raisin Cookie
- ✓ White Chip Macadamia Cookie
- ✓ Chocolate Chip with M&M Cookie
- ✓ Snickerdoodle Cookie

Traditional

Au Bon Pain

Entrées

- ✓ Mayan Chicken Harvest Rice Bowl with brown or white rice

Salad

- ✓ BBQ Beef Salad
- ✓ Egg and Cucumber Salad
- ✓ Potato Bacon Salad
- ✓ Red Bliss Potato Salad
- ✓ Tomato and Cucumber Salad
- ✓ Tomato, Green Bean and Almond Salad
- ✓ Tuna Salad
- ✓ Watermelon and Feta Salad
- ✓ Chef's Salad
- ✓ Greek Salad
- ✓ Mediterranean Chicken Salad

Dressings, Sauces, and Spreads

- ✓ All sauces, condiments, and spreads

Soup

- ✓ Black Bean Soup
- ✓ Curried Rice and Lentil Soup
- ✓ Fresh Moroccan Tomato Lentil
- ✓ Garden Vegetable

- ✓ Gazpacho
- ✓ Portuguese Kale
- ✓ Potato Cheese
- ✓ Southwest Tortilla
- ✓ Beef Chili
- ✓ Vegetarian Chili
- ✓ Tuscan white bean

Sides

- ✓ White rice
- ✓ Brown rice
- ✓ Roasted Potatoes
- ✓ Sausage with Pepper and Onions
- ✓ Scrambled Eggs
- ✓ Oatmeal
- ✓ Apple Cinnamon Oatmeal
- ✓ Hummus and Cucumber Portion
- ✓ Mozzarella and Tomato Portion
- ✓ Turkey, Asparagus, Cranberry, Chutney and Gorgonzola Portion

Snacks and Dessert

- ✓ All yogurts
- ✓ Chocolate Covered Strawberry
- ✓ Dark Chocolate Covered Raisins
- ✓ Fresh Grapes
- ✓ Fresh Pineapples
- ✓ Fresh Watermelon
- ✓ Fruit Cup
- ✓ Mixed Nuts

- ✓ Muesli
- ✓ Sugar Free Cinnamon Buttons
- ✓ Turkish Apricots
- ✓ Apples, Blue Cheese and Cranberries Portion

Boston Market

Entrée

- ✓ Roasted Turkey Breast
- ✓ Rotisserie Chicken

Sides

- ✓ Butternut Squash
- ✓ Cinnamon Apples
- ✓ Coleslaw
- ✓ Creamed Spinach
- ✓ Fresh Steamed Vegetables
- ✓ Garlic Dill New Potatoes
- ✓ Mashed Potatoes
- ✓ Sweet Corn
- ✓ Loaded Mashed Potatoes
- ✓ Mediterranean Green Beans
- ✓ Garlicky Spinach

Salads

- ✓ Southwest Santa Fe

Sauces

- ✓ Frank's Sweet Heat
- ✓ Honey Habanero
- ✓ Island Mojo

Chicken

Chick Fil A

Below is a list of their menu items that may fit your
gluten-free diet. Some ingredients such as spices and
natural flavors may be proprietary; therefore, Chick
Fil A may not have the source listed for those items.
Chick Fil A recommends you review this list with your
physician before consuming any of the products listed
below, or any other item on our menu.

Entree

- ✓ Chick-fil-A Chargrilled Chicken Filet
- ✓ Chick-fil-A Chargrilled Chicken Garden
  Salad
- ✓ Chick-fil-A Chargrilled Chicken & Fruit
  Salad
- ✓ Tortilla Strips

Sides

- ✓ Fruit Cup
- ✓ Side Salad
- ✓ Cole Slaw
- ✓ Carrot & Raisin Salad
- ✓ Chick-fil-A Waffle Potato Fries
- ✓ Yogurt Parfait
- ✓ Breakfast
- ✓ Bacon slice
- ✓ Egg

- ✓ Sausage patty
- ✓ American cheese slice
- ✓ Hash Browns

Desserts

- ✓ Icedream
- ✓ Chocolate Syrup
- ✓ Blueberry Topping

Beverages

- ✓ All Beverages

Dipping Sauces and Dressings

- ✓ Barbecue Sauce
- ✓ Honey Mustard Sauce
- ✓ Honey Roasted BBQ Sauce
- ✓ Polynesian Sauce
- ✓ Buttermilk Ranch Sauce
- ✓ Chick-fil-A Buffalo Sauce
- ✓ Spicy Dressing
- ✓ Blue Cheese Dressing
- ✓ Buttermilk Ranch Dressing
- ✓ Thousand Island Dressing
- ✓ Light Italian Dressing
- ✓ Fat Free Dijon Honey Mustard Dressing
- ✓ Caesar Dressing
- ✓ Reduced Fat Raspberry Vinaigrette Dressing

- ✓ Reduced Fat Berry Balsamic Vinaigrette Dressing
- ✓ Chick-fil-A Sauce
- ✓ Condiments
- ✓ Ketchup
- ✓ Mustard
- ✓ Mayonnaise
- ✓ Apple Jelly
- ✓ Grape Jelly
- ✓ Mixed Fruit Jelly

Kentucky Fried Chicken (KFC)

- ✓ Three bean salad
- ✓ House Side Salad without Dressing
- ✓ Green beans
- ✓ Corn on the Cobb
- ✓ Sweet Cornel Corn
- ✓ Potato Salad
- ✓ Sargento Light String Cheese

Dipping sauce and Dressings

- ✓ Honey Barbeque Sandwich Sauce
- ✓ Honey Mustard BBQ Sauce
- ✓ Pepper Mayonnaise
- ✓ Spicy Mayonnaise
- ✓ KFC Signature Sauce Dipping Cup
- ✓ Spicy Chipotle Dipping Sauce
- ✓ Creamy Ranch Dipping Sauce
- ✓ HBBQ Dipping Sauce

- ✓ Tartar Sauce
- ✓ Honey Sauce
- ✓ Colonel's Buttery Spread
- ✓ Heinz Buttermilk Ranch Dressing
- ✓ Hidden Valley The Original Ranch Fat Free Dressing
- ✓ Marzetti Light Italian Dressing

Popeyes

- ✓ Red beans
- ✓ Cole slaw
- ✓ Corn on the cob (at participating locations)
- ✓ Cajun rice

Raising Canes

Here's what Raising Cane's told me about their gluten free selection so hopefully this helps you out.

"Raising Cane's® the breading for our chicken and our toast does contain gluten. The coleslaw, Cane's Sauce, and fries are all gluten free; however, due to the fact that our chicken and fries sometimes share fryers during our peak times, we cannot guarantee our fries to be gluten free.

In the past, we have accommodated guests with dairy and egg allergies by cooking "naked" chicken fingers.

This is not a frequent occurrence and is done at the discretion of the management at the location.

If you do decide to visit any of our locations, please ask for the manager on duty and notify them of the dairy allergy so that they may best accommodate you. Thank you for allowing us to serve you and we look forward to the next time."

Entrees

- ✓ Chicken Fingers without breading

Sides

- ✓ Cole Slaw
- ✓ Fries

Sauces and Condiments

- ✓ Cane's Sauce

Seafood

Captain D's

Entrees

- ✓ Classic Catfish
- ✓ Wild Alaskan Salmon
- ✓ Wild Alaskan Salmon Salad
- ✓ Shrimp Skewers
- ✓ Premium Shrimp
- ✓ Seasoned Tilapia
- ✓ Shrimp Scampi

Sides

- ✓ Brocolli
- ✓ Sliced Cheese
- ✓ Corn on the Cobb
- ✓ Green Beans
- ✓ Side Salad
- ✓ Roasted Red Potatoes
- ✓ Baked Potatoes

Sauces and Condiments

- ✓ Sweet Chili Sauce
- ✓ Tartar Sauce
- ✓ Blue Cheese Dressing
- ✓ Honey Mustard Dressing
- ✓ Ranch Dressing
- ✓ Thousand Island Dressing

- ✓ Mayo
- ✓ Cocktail Sauce

Long John Silver

Entrée

- ✓ Grilled Pacific Salmon
- ✓ Shrimp Scampi
- ✓ Freshside Grille Salmon Entrée
- ✓ Freshside Grille Shrimp Scampi Entrée

Sides

- ✓ Cole Slaw
- ✓ Corn Cobbette without Butter Oil
- ✓ Corn Cobbette with Butter Oil
- ✓ Rice
- ✓ Vegetable Medley

Condiments

- ✓ Cocktail Sauce
- ✓ Tartar Sauce
- ✓ Baja Sauce
- ✓ Louisiana Hot Sauce
- ✓ Ketchup

Desserts

- ✓ Iceflow Lemonade
- ✓ Iceflow Strawberry Lemonade

Hispanic and Southwest

Baja Fresh

- ✓ Baja Tacos made with corn tortillas
- ✓ Any "Bare style" burrito
- ✓ Baja Ensalada with choice of steak, chicken, grilled shrimp or Mahi Mahi, grilled vegetables, carnitas, rice, and both varieties of beans
- ✓ All dressings
- ✓ All salsas

Chipotle

- ✓ Crispy Taco Shell
- ✓ Cilantro Lime Rice
- ✓ Black Beans
- ✓ Pinto Beans
- ✓ Fajita Vegetables
- ✓ Barbacoa
- ✓ Chicken
- ✓ Camitas
- ✓ Steak
- ✓ Tomato Salsa
- ✓ Corn Salsa
- ✓ Red Tomatillo Salso
- ✓ Cheese

- ✓ Sour Cream
- ✓ Guacamole
- ✓ Romaine Lettuce
- ✓ Chips
- ✓ Vinaigrette
- ✓ Soft Corn Tortilla
- ✓ Breakfast Eggs
- ✓ Breakfast Relish
- ✓ Breakfast Chorizo
- ✓ Breakfast Potatoes

Del Taco

- ✓ Plain hamburger patty
- ✓ Cheddar cheese
- ✓ Spicy Jack Cheese
- ✓ Rice
- ✓ Red Sauce
- ✓ Green Sauce
- ✓ Taco Shells
- ✓ Tortilla Shells
- ✓ Lettuce
- ✓ Tomato
- ✓ Onion
- ✓ Vanilla Shake

El Pollo Loco

- ✓ Pinto Beans
- ✓ Refried beans
- ✓ Cotija cheese
- ✓ Mixed Vegetables

- ✓ Corn tortillas
- ✓ Flame grilled Mexican chicken
- ✓ Avocado Salsa
- ✓ Flan
- ✓ All drinks and beverages

Moe's Southwest Grill

Proteins

- ✓ Chicken
- ✓ Steak
- ✓ Ground Beef
- ✓ Pork
- ✓ Tofu
- ✓ Fish

Beans

- ✓ Black beans
- ✓ Pinto Beans

Toppings and Extras

- ✓ Black olives
- ✓ Cheese
- ✓ Chipotle ranch
- ✓ Cucumbers
- ✓ Guacamole
- ✓ Jalapenos
- ✓ Lettuce

- ✓ Cheese (Queso)
- ✓ Rice
- ✓ Salsa (Kaiser and El Guapo)
- ✓ Sour Cream
- ✓ Southwest Vinaigrette
- ✓ Veggies
- ✓ Tomatillo Salsa
- ✓ Pico de Gallo
- ✓ Corn Pico de Gallo
- ✓ Hard Rock 'N Roll Sauce

Qdoba

Entrée

- ✓ Soft White Corn Tortilla
- ✓ Cilantro Lime Rice
- ✓ Black Beans
- ✓ Pork
- ✓ Chicken
- ✓ Ground Sirloin
- ✓ Seasoned Shredded Beef
- ✓ Flat Iron Steak
- ✓ Chorizo
- ✓ Eggs
- ✓ Tortilla Soup

Salsas and Dressings

- ✓ Poblano Pesto
- ✓ 3 Cheese Queso
- ✓ Ranchera
- ✓ Guacamole

- ✓ Lite Sour Cream
- ✓ Fat Free Ranch Dressing
- ✓ Fat Free Picante Ranch Dressing
- ✓ Cilantro Lime Vinaigrette

Taco Bell

- ✓ Pintos 'n Cheese
- ✓ Mexican Rice
- ✓ Tostada

Taco John's

Entrees

- ✓ Crispy Taco
- ✓ Crispy Taco with Cheese
- ✓ Super Nachos
- ✓ Super Potato Oles

Sides

- ✓ Nachos
- ✓ Potato Oles
- ✓ Chili w/o Crackers
- ✓ Chili w/o Crackers and Cheese
- ✓ Refried Beans

Sauces and Condiments

- ✓ Mild Sauce
- ✓ Hot Sauce

- ✓ Super Hot Sauce
- ✓ Pico de Gallo
- ✓ Salsa
- ✓ Sour Cream X
- ✓ Guacamole
- ✓ Nacho Cheese Sauce
- ✓ House Dressing
- ✓ Ranch Dressing
- ✓ Bacon Ranch Dressing
- ✓ Creamy Italian Dressing

Taco Time

Entrée

- ✓ Crispy Ground Beef Taco with or without sour cream
- ✓ Ground Beef Enchilada

Sides

- ✓ Chips
- ✓ Cheddar Fries
- ✓ Mexi-Fries
- ✓ Mexi-Rice
- ✓ Refritos with Chips
- ✓ Sauces and Dressings
- ✓ Sour Cream
- ✓ Guacamole
- ✓ Salsa Fresca
- ✓ Salsa Nuevo
- ✓ Salsa Verde

- ✓ Chipotle Ranch Dressing
- ✓ Ranch Dressing
- ✓ Thousand Island Dressing

Sandwiches, Deli, and Salads

Blimpie

Individual Menu Items

- ✓ Bacon
- ✓ Buffalo Chicken
- ✓ Cappacola
- ✓ Grilled Chicken Strips
- ✓ Corned Beef
- ✓ Ham
- ✓ Pastrami
- ✓ Pepperoni
- ✓ Philly Steak & Onion
- ✓ Prosciuttini
- ✓ Roast Beef
- ✓ Salami
- ✓ Seafood Salad
- ✓ Tuna
- ✓ Turkey
- ✓ American Yellow & White
- ✓ Smoked Cheddar
- ✓ Shredded Mild Cheddar
- ✓ Shredded Parmesan
- ✓ Provolone
- ✓ Swiss

Salads

- ✓ Antipasto

- ✓ Buffalo Chicken
- ✓ Chef
- ✓ Chicken Caesar
- ✓ Tuna
- ✓ Ultimate Club
- ✓ Garden
- ✓ Cole Slaw
- ✓ Northwest Potato
- ✓ Potato

Soups

- ✓ Captain's Corn Chowder
- ✓ Cream of Broccoli with Cheese
- ✓ Cream of Potato
- ✓ Grande Chili w/ith Bean & Beef X
- ✓ Pilgrim Turkey Vegetables with Rice

Chips

- ✓ Cheddar Sour Cream Lays
- ✓ Cheetos, Crunchy
- ✓ Doritos Cooler Ranch
- ✓ Fritos
- ✓ BBQ Lays
- ✓ Lays Potato Baked
- ✓ Lays Potato Regular

Dressings and Sauces

- ✓ All sauces and dressings

Charley's Grilled Subs

Entrées without Toasted Bun

- ✓ Philly Cheesesteak
- ✓ Philly Steak Deluxe
- ✓ BBQ Cheddar
- ✓ Bacon 3 Cheese
- ✓ Sicilian Steak
- ✓ Mushroom Swiss Steak
- ✓ Philly Steak and Bleu
- ✓ Philly Chicken
- ✓ Chicken California
- ✓ Chicken Buffalo
- ✓ Chicken Teriyaki
- ✓ Chicken Cordon Bleu
- ✓ Chicken Bacon Club
- ✓ Turkey Cheddar Melt
- ✓ Philly Ham and Swiss
- ✓ Italian Deli
- ✓ Philly Veggie

Sides

- ✓ Fries
- ✓ Ranch Bacon Fries
- ✓ Cheddar Bacon Fries
- ✓ Cheddar Fries
- ✓ Ultimate fries

Beverages

- ✓ All beverages

Salad

- ✓ Grilled Chicken Salad
- ✓ Chicken Teriyaki Salad
- ✓ Buffalo Chicken Salad
- ✓ Grilled Steak Salad
- ✓ Fresh Garden Salad

Breakfast

- ✓ Two eggs scrambled
- ✓ Ham Omelet
- ✓ Bacon Omelet
- ✓ Sausage Omelet
- ✓ Veggie Omelet
- ✓ Western Omelet
- ✓ Egg and Cheese Sandwich
- ✓ Bacon, Egg and Cheese Sandwich
- ✓ Sausage, Egg and Cheese Sandwich
- ✓ Steak, Egg and Cheese Sandwich
- ✓ Hash Browns

Jason's Deli

Build Your Own Sandwich

- ✓ Gluten-free bread
- ✓ Hot pastrami
- ✓ Hot corned beef
- ✓ Roast beef
- ✓ Oven roasted turkey breast
- ✓ Smoked turkey breast

- ✓ Premium ham
- ✓ Chicken salad made wlth
- ✓ almonds & pineapple
- ✓ Tuna salad
- ✓ Hard salami
- ✓ Natural grilled chicken breast
- ✓ Yellow mustard
- ✓ Organic stone ground mustard
- ✓ Mayonnaise
- ✓ Smoked red pepper-cilantro aioli
- ✓ Leo's Italian dressing
- ✓ Balsamic Vinegar (bottle)
- ✓ Extra virgin olive oil
- ✓ Lettuce
- ✓ Tomato
- ✓ Organic field greens
- ✓ Organic spinach
- ✓ Purple onion rings
- ✓ Italian peppers
- ✓ Our family recipe pico de gallo
- ✓ Our family recipe guacamole
- ✓ Sliced avocado
- ✓ Oven roasted herb tomatoes
- ✓ Swiss
- ✓ American
- ✓ Cheddar
- ✓ Jalapeño pepper jack
- ✓ Provolone

Soups

- ✓ Vegetarian Tomato Basil
- ✓ Organic Vegetable Soup
- ✓ Fire-Roasted Tortilla
- ✓ Red Beans & Rice with sausage

Salads and Salad Bar Toppings

- ✓ Big Chef
- ✓ Nutty Mixed Up Salad
- ✓ Chicken Club Salad
- ✓ Lettuce
- ✓ Organic field greens
- ✓ Organic spinach
- ✓ Cauliflower
- ✓ Grape tomatoes
- ✓ Broccoli
- ✓ Mushrooms
- ✓ Organic baby carrots
- ✓ Red bell pepper rings
- ✓ Yellow bell pepper rings
- ✓ Purple onion rings
- ✓ Cucumber slices
- ✓ Sprouts
- ✓ Green olives
- ✓ Kalamata olives
- ✓ Artichokes
- ✓ Italian peppers
- ✓ Hard boiled eggs
- ✓ Bacon bits

- ✓ Organic apple slices
- ✓ Mixed fruit and yogurt
- ✓ Cottage cheese
- ✓ Feta
- ✓ Shredded asiago
- ✓ Shredded cheddar
- ✓ Roasted red pepper hummus
- ✓ American potato salad
- ✓ Coleslaw
- ✓ Walnut cranberry trail mix
- ✓ Chocolate mousse

Dressings

- ✓ Bleu Cheese
- ✓ Low fat Honey Mustard
- ✓ Our family recipe Ranch
- ✓ Low fat Ranch
- ✓ Leo's Italian
- ✓ Organic Raspberry Vinaigrette
- ✓ Creamy Caesar
- ✓ Thousand Island
- ✓ Organic Country French
- ✓ Extra Virgin Olive Oil (bottle)
- ✓ Organic Balsamic Vinegar

Potatoes

- ✓ Texas Style Spud
- ✓ Pollo Mexicano
- ✓ The Plain Jane

Sides

- ✓ Chips or baked chips & pickle
- ✓ Organic blue corn tortilla chips & salsa
- ✓ Organic blue corn tortilla chips &
- ✓ Roasted red pepper hummus
- ✓ Organic blue corn tortilla chips &guacamole
- ✓ American potato salad
- ✓ Steamed veggies
- ✓ Fresh fruit & creamy fruit dip

Desserts

- ✓ Chocolate or vanilla ice cream with no cone
- ✓ Chocolate syrup topping

Kid's Menu

- ✓ Grilled Cheese on gluten-free bread
- ✓ Hot dog on gluten-free bun
- ✓ Organic Peanut Butter and Jelly on gluten-free bread
- ✓ Ham and Cheese on gluten-free bread
- ✓ Turkey and Cheese on gluten-free bread

Panera Bread

Salads

- ✓ Greek Salad Caesar Salad (without croutons)
- ✓ Grilled Chicken
- ✓ Caesar Salad (without croutons)
- ✓ Asian Sesame Chicken Salad (without Won Ton noodles)
- ✓ Classic Cafe Salad
- ✓ Fuji Apple Chicken Salad (G)
- ✓ Chopped Chicken Cobb Salad (G)
- ✓ Strawberry Poppyseed Chicken Salad
- ✓ Tomato and Mozzarella Salad (without croutons)
- ✓ BBQ Chopped Chicken Salad
- ✓ Fruit Cup – Watermelon
- ✓ Seasonal Mixed Fruit Cup

Salad Dressings

- ✓ Balsamic Vinaigrette
- ✓ Caesar
- ✓ Greek
- ✓ Poppyseed Dressing
- ✓ Asian Sesame Vinaigrette
- ✓ White Balsamic Vinaigrette
- ✓ BBQ Ranch
- ✓ Light Buttermilk Ranch

Soups

- ✓ Low Fat Vegetarian Black Bean
- ✓ Creamy Tomato (without croutons)

Beverages

- ✓ Coffee
- ✓ Juice, both apple and orange
- ✓ Lemonade
- ✓ Milk
- ✓ Soda, fountain and bottled
- ✓ Tea, regular and Chai Tea
- ✓ All lattes & Frozen beverages
- ✓ Low-fat Strawberry Smoothie
- ✓ Low-Fat Black Cherry Smoothie
- ✓ Low-Fat Mango Smoothie
- ✓ Low-fat Wild Berry Smoothie
- ✓ Frozen Strawberry Lemonade
- ✓ Frozen Lemonade
- ✓ Hot Chocolate

Sides

- ✓ Panera Bread Potato Chips

SaladWorks

Salads, Toppings, and Dressing

- ✓ Bacon
- ✓ Blue Cheese Crumbles
- ✓ Chicken

- ✓ Corn blend
- ✓ Blue Cheese Dressing
- ✓ Dressing Creamy Italian
- ✓ Lite Ranch Dressing
- ✓ FF Balsamic Dressing
- ✓ FF Caesar Dressing
- ✓ FF Honey Dressing
- ✓ French Dressing
- ✓ Green Goddess Dressing
- ✓ Italian Vinaigrette Dressing
- ✓ Lite Raspberry Dressing
- ✓ Parm Peppercorn Dressing
- ✓ Ranch Dressing
- ✓ Russian Dressing
- ✓ Balsamic Vinaigrette Dressing
- ✓ Lemon Capri Dressing
- ✓ Yogurt Caesar Dressing
- ✓ Yogurt Italian Dressing
- ✓ Eggs/Egg Whites
- ✓ Fire Roasted Red Pepper
- ✓ Grated Parmesan
- ✓ Ham
- ✓ Mandarin Oranges
- ✓ Monterey Jack
- ✓ Mozzarella
- ✓ Olives
- ✓ Pepperoni
- ✓ Sun Dried Tomatoes
- ✓ Sunflower Seeds
- ✓ Swiss Cheese
- ✓ Tofu

- ✓ Tortilla Strips
- ✓ Tuna
- ✓ Turkey
- ✓ Walnuts
- ✓ Provolone Cheese

Soups

- ✓ Beef Chili
- ✓ Broccoli Cheddar
- ✓ Chicken Chili
- ✓ Chicken Tortilla

Subway

Salads

- ✓ Buffalo Chicken
- ✓ Chicken and Bacon Ranch
- ✓ Cold Cut Combo
- ✓ Ham (Black Forest)
- ✓ Italian BMT
- ✓ Oven Roasted Chicken with Chicken Strips
- ✓ Roast Beef
- ✓ Tuna
- ✓ Turkey Breast
- ✓ Turkey Breast and Ham
- ✓ Spicy Italian
- ✓ Subway Club
- ✓ Veggie Delight

Meat, Poultry, Seafood, and Eggs

- ✓ Bacon Strips
- ✓ Oven Roasted Chicken
- ✓ Chicken Strips (plain)
- ✓ Cold Cut Combo Meats
- ✓ Egg (Regular) Omelet
- ✓ Egg (White) Omelet
- ✓ Ham (Black Forest)
- ✓ Italian BMT Meats
- ✓ Roast Beef
- ✓ Steak
- ✓ Tuna
- ✓ Turkey Breast

Cheese

- ✓ American Cheese
- ✓ Cheddar Cheese
- ✓ Monterey Cheddar Cheese, Shredded
- ✓ Mozzarella Cheese, Shredded
- ✓ Parmesan Cheese
- ✓ Pepper Jack Cheese
- ✓ Provolone Cheese
- ✓ Swiss Cheese

Condiments and Dressing

- ✓ Buffalo Sauce
- ✓ Chipotle Southwest Sauce
- ✓ Honey Mustard Sauce
- ✓ Light Mayonnaise/Regular Mayonnaise
- ✓ Mustard (Yellow and Deli Brown)
- ✓ Oil

- ✓ Ranch Dressing
- ✓ Red Wine Vinaigrette
- ✓ Sweet Onion Sauce (Contains Poppy Seeds)
- ✓ Vinegar

Vegetables

- ✓ Banana Peppers
- ✓ Jalapenos
- ✓ Olives
- ✓ Pickles
- ✓ Vegetables, Fresh

Foreign

Noodles & Company

NOTE....BE SURE TO ASK FOR RICE NOODLES

Noodle Entrée

- ✓ Pad Thai with rice noodles
- ✓ Penne Rosa with rice noodles
- ✓ Pasta Fresca with rice noodles
- ✓ Whole Grain Tuscan Linguine with rice noodles
- ✓ Spaghetti with Marinara Sauce
- ✓ Buttered Noodles
- ✓ Sautéed Beef
- ✓ Braised Beef
- ✓ Sautéed Shrimp

Salad

- ✓ Chinese Chopped Salad with no wonton strips
- ✓ The Mediterranean Salad with no cavatappi noodles
- ✓ Cucumber Tomato Salad
- ✓ Tossed Green Salad with Balsamic
- ✓ Tossed Green Salad with Fat Free Asian

Pollo Tropical

Entrée

- ✓ Chicken
- ✓ Pork
-   Shrimp

Sides

- ✓ Corn
- ✓ Red beans
- ✓ Cheddar Cheese

Desserts

- ✓ Flan
- ✓ Guava Cheesecake

Sauces

- ✓ Curry Mustard Sauce

Drinks

- ✓ All drinks and beverages

Desserts and Drinks

Baskin Robins

Hand Scooped
- ✓ Premium Churned Light Cappuccino Chip
- ✓ Premium Churned Reduced Fat, No Sugar Added Caramel Truffle Turtle
- ✓ Super Soldier Swirl
- ✓ Firehouse
- ✓ Toffee Pecan Crunch
- ✓ White Caramel Chocolate Frozen Yogurt
- ✓ Fat Free Vanilla Frozen Yogurt
- ✓ Watermelon Chip
- ✓ Pink Grapefruit Sorbet
- ✓ Premium Churned Reduced Fat Pineapple Coconut
- ✓ Premium Churned Reduced Chocolate Overload
- ✓ Premium Churned Reduced Butter Almond Crunch
- ✓ Tax Crunch
- ✓ Cotton Candy
- ✓ Jamoca
- ✓ Mint Chocolate Chip
- ✓ Jamoca Almond Fudge
- ✓ Mint Chocolate Chip
- ✓ Jamoca Almond Fudge
- ✓ Lemon Custard

- ✓ Pistachio Almond
- ✓ Oregon Black Berry
- ✓ Baseball Nut
- ✓ Pumpkin Pie
- ✓ Egg Nog
- ✓ Nutty Coconut
- ✓ Bananas 'n Strawberries
- ✓ Pralines 'n Cream
- ✓ Quarterback Crunch
- ✓ Gold Medal Ribbon
- ✓ Banana Nut
- ✓ Chocolate Mousse Royal
- ✓ Cherries Jubilee
- ✓ World Class Chocolate
- ✓ Winter White Chocolate
- ✓ Reese's Peanut Butter Cup
- ✓ Snickers
- ✓ Chocolate
- ✓ Peanut Butter 'n Chocolate
- ✓ Chocolate Chip
- ✓ Very Berry Strawberry
- ✓ Rum Raisin
- ✓ Chocolate Almond
- ✓ Rocky Road
- ✓ Vanilla
- ✓ Old Fashioned Butter Pecan
- ✓ Love Potion #31
- ✓ Creole Cream Cheese
- ✓ Chocolate Fudge
- ✓ Orange Sherbet
- ✓ Rock 'n Pop Swirl

- ✓ Wild 'n Reckless Sherbet
- ✓ Splish Splash Sherbet
- ✓ Rainbow Sherbet
- ✓ Daiquiri Ice
- ✓ Lemon Sorbet
- ✓ Tropical Ice
- ✓ Watermelon Chip

Soft Serve

- ✓ Strawberry Fruit Cream
- ✓ Peach Passion Fruit Cream
- ✓ Reese's Mini Parfait
- ✓ Strawberry 'n Almonds
- ✓ Vanilla
- ✓ Reese's Peanut Butter Cup
- ✓ Heath 31°
- ✓ Strawberry Banana Below 31°
- ✓ Mango Fruit Cream
- ✓ Hot Fudge Sundae
- ✓ Strawberry
- ✓ Caramel Sundae
- ✓ Butterfinger
- ✓ Jamoca Almond Fudge

Sundaes

- ✓ Two-scoop
- ✓ Classic Banana Split
- ✓ Banana Royale
- ✓ Reese's Peanut Butter Cup

✓ Snickers

Beverages

✓ Cappuccino Blast Nonfat
✓ Freeze with Orange Sherbet
✓ Ice Cream Soda with Vanilla
✓ Ice Cream Float with Vanilla and Root Beer
✓ Chocolate Chip Shake
✓ Peach Passion Banana Fruit Blast Smoothie
✓ Peach Passion Fruit Blast
✓ Raspberry Chip Shake with premium
   Churned Light Raspberry Chip ice cream
✓ Chocolate Shake
✓ Strawberry Banana Fruit Blast Smoothie
✓ Strawberry Citrus Fruit Blast
✓ Cappuccino Blast Original
✓ Cappuccino Blast Nonfat
✓ Cappuccino Blast Mocha
✓ Vanilla Shake
✓ Chocolate Shake with Vanilla ice cream
✓ Chocolate Shake with Chocolate ice cream
✓ Cappuccino Blast Turtle
✓ Wild Mango Fruit Blast
✓ Strawberry Shake
✓ Wild Mango Fruit Blast
✓ Mango Fruit Blast Smoothie
✓ Cappuccino Blast Original
✓ Mint Chocolate Chip Shake
✓ Cappuccino Blast Caramel
✓ Cappuccino Blast with Soft Serve

Dunkin Donuts

- ✓ All coffee
- ✓ All Beverages

Jamba Juice

Drinks and Smoothies

- ✓ 3G Charger Boost
- ✓ Acai Super-Antioxidant
- ✓ Antioxidant Power Boost
- ✓ Apple 'n Greens
- ✓ Banana Berry
- ✓ Berry Fulfilling
- ✓ Berry UpBeet
- ✓ Blackberry Bliss
- ✓ Caribbean Passion
- ✓ Carrot Juice
- ✓ Chocolate Moo'd
- ✓ Classic Hot Chocolate
- ✓ Coffee Craze
- ✓ Five Fruit Frenzy
- ✓ Flax and Fiber Boost
- ✓ Immunity Boost
- ✓ Mango Mantra
- ✓ Mango-a-go-go
- ✓ Matcha Energy Shot-Orange Juice
- ✓ Matcha Energy Shot-Soymilk

- ✓ Matcha Green Tea Blast
- ✓ Mega Mango
- ✓ Mocha Mojo
- ✓ Orange Carrot Karma
- ✓ Orange Dream Machine
- ✓ Orange Juice
- ✓ Orange-A-Peel
- ✓ Organic African Nectar
- ✓ Organic Breakfast
- ✓ Organic Detox Infusion
- ✓ Organic Earl Grey
- ✓ Organic Green Drago
- ✓ Organic House Blend
- ✓ Organic House Blend Decaf
- ✓ Organic Spring Jasmine
- ✓ Original Spiced Chai
- ✓ Peach Perfection
- ✓ Peach Pleasure
- ✓ Peanut Butter Moo'd
- ✓ Pomegranate Paradise
- ✓ Pomegranate Pick-Me-Up
- ✓ Protein Berry Workout
- ✓ Pumpkin Smash
- ✓ Razzmatazz
- ✓ Soy Protein Boost
- ✓ Strawberries Wild
- ✓ Strawberry Nirvana
- ✓ Strawberry Surf Rider
- ✓ Strawberry Whirl
- ✓ The Coldbuster
- ✓ Whey Protein Boost

Starbucks

Hot Breakfast

- ✓ Starbucks Perfect Oatmel
- ✓ Brown Sugar topping for Starbucks Perfect Oatmeal
- ✓ Dried Fruit topping for Starbucks Perfect Oatmeal
- ✓ Nut Medley topping for Starbucks Perfect Oatmeal

Salads

- ✓ Deluxe Fruit Blend

Yogurt Parfaits

- ✓ Dark Cherry Yogurt Parfait
- ✓ Strawberry and Blueberry Yogurt Parfait
- ✓ Greek Yogurt Parfait

Bakery

- ✓ Marshmallow Dream Bar

Drinks and Beverages

- ✓ Starbucks DoubleShot Energy+...all flavors
- ✓ Starbucks Bottled Frappucino Coffee Drink...all flavors
- ✓ Bold Pick of the Day

- ✓ Café Misto
- ✓ Clover Brewed Coffee
- ✓ Coffee Traveler
- ✓ Decaf Pike Place Roast
- ✓ Iced Coffee
- ✓ Iced Coffee with Milk
- ✓ Pike Place Roast
- ✓ Hot Chocolate
- ✓ Peppermint Hot Chocolate
- ✓ Salted Caramel Hot Chocolate
- ✓ White Hot Chocolate
- ✓ Café Vanilla Frappuccino
- ✓ All Expresso
- ✓ All Vivanno Smoothies
- ✓ All Tazo Teas
- ✓ All Kid's Drinks

Frappuccino Blended Beverages

- ✓ Café Vanilla
- ✓ Caramel
- ✓ Caramel Brulee
- ✓ Cinnamon Dolce
- ✓ Cinnamon Crème
- ✓ Coconut Crème
- ✓ Coffee
- ✓ Double Chocolate Chip
- ✓ Espresso
- ✓ Extra Coffee
- ✓ Java Chip
- ✓ Mocha Coconut

- ✓ Mocha
- ✓ Peppermint Mocha
- ✓ Soy Strawberries Crème
- ✓ Tazo Chai Crème
- ✓ Tazo Green Teal Crème
- ✓ Vanilla Bean Crème
- ✓ White Chocolate Crème
- ✓ White Chocolate Mocha

TCBY

Toppings

- ✓ All fruit toppings
- ✓ Caramel topping
- ✓ Hot fudge topping
- ✓ Chocolate topping
- ✓ Marshmallow topping
- ✓ Whipped topping
- ✓ Peanut Butter topping

Soft Serve

- ✓ Vanilla
- ✓ Chocolate
- ✓ Classic Tart
- ✓ Dutch Chocolate
- ✓ Coffee
- ✓ Strawberry
- ✓ Golden Vanilla
- ✓ Old Fashioned Vanilla
- ✓ Fat Free Mountain Black Berry
- ✓ White Chocolate Macadamia Nut

- ✓ White Chocolate Mouse
- ✓ Mango Sorbet
- ✓ Kiwi Strawberry Sorbet
- ✓ Orange Sorbet
- ✓ Ruby Red Grapefruit Sorbet

Hand Scooped

- ✓ Blueberries and Cream
- ✓ Butter pecan Perfection
- ✓ Chocolate Chocolate
- ✓ Mint Chocolate Chunk
- ✓ Cotton Candy
- ✓ Mocha Almond
- ✓ Peaches and Cream
- ✓ Peanut Butter Delight
- ✓ Pralines and Cream
- ✓ Vanilla Bean
- ✓ Vanilla Chocolate Chunk
- ✓ Very Berry Strawberry
- ✓ White Chocolate Mouse
- ✓ Rainbow Cream
- ✓ Psychedelic Sorbet

Adam's Top Picks

The Best Restaurants for Gluten-Free Eating

- ✓ Jason's Deli
- ✓ Au Bon Pain
- ✓ Chick Fil A
- ✓ Chipotle
- ✓ Qdoba
- ✓ SaladWorks
- ✓ Subway
- ✓ Starbucks
- ✓ TCBY
- ✓ Baskin Robins

Made in the USA
Lexington, KY
27 February 2013